Essentials in Hospice and Palliative Care:
A RESOURCE FOR NURSING ASSISTANTS

INSTRUCTOR'S GUIDE

Katherine Murray
RN, BSN, MA, FT, CHPCN(C)

Life and Death Matters
Victoria, BC

Life & Death Matters

www.lifeanddeathmatters.ca

Published by Life and Death Matters, Victoria, BC, Canada
www.lifeanddeathmatters.ca

Illustrations by Joanne Thomson
Editing by Ann-Marie Gilbert
Design by Greg Glover

Printed in U.S.A.

Library and Archives Canada Cataloguing in Publication

Murray, Katherine, 1957–, author
        Essentials in hospice and palliative care. Instructor's guide : a
resource for nursing assistants / Katherine Murray, RN, BSN, MA,
CHPCN(C).

A study guide to: Essentials in hospice and palliative care : a resource
        for nursing assistants / Katherine Murray, RN, BSN, MA,
        CHPCN(C). — Victoria, BC : Life and Death Matters, 2015.
ISBN 978-1-926923-10-9 (paperback)

        1. Hospice care--Study and teaching. 2. Palliative treatment—Study
and teaching. 3. Hospice nurses. 4. Nurses' aides. I. Title.

RT87.T45M87 2015 Suppl.   616.02'9071   C2015-902933-3

Disclaimer

This book is intended only as a resource of general education on the subject matter. Every effort has been made to en-sure the accuracy of the information it contains; however, there is no guarantee that the information will remain current beyond the date of publication. The information and techniques provided in this book should be used in consultation with qualified medical health professionals and should not be considered a replacement, substitute, or alternative for their guidance, assessment, or treatment. The author and publisher accept no responsibility or liability with respect to any person or entity for loss or damage or any other problem caused or alleged to be caused directly or indirectly by information contained in this book.

Contents

Preface

Several years ago I had the privilege of working with a team of hospice and palliative care leaders to address the question, "How do we prepare the workforce to care for the coming tsunami of dying people?" The question we asked as a group became a personal quest: "How can I help prepare front line caregivers to care for the coming tsunami of dying people?"

My purpose in writing the text *Essentials in Hospice and Palliative Care: A Resource for Nursing Assistants* and companion workbook was to help nursing assistants become more confident and competent in providing excellent and compassionate care for the dying person and their family.

My goals for developing teaching resources, including videos, PowerPoint™ presentations, podcasts, and this instructor's guide were to assist instructors (you) in delivering excellent education, within core curriculum, and, I hope, decrease the preparation time required to teach the content. These resources can also be used in workplace education to build on the basic concepts taught in core curriculum.

The instructor's guide *is not* a manual on how to teach. *It is* a resource that provides strategies for teaching this content and identifies relevant content in each of the related resources. Many instructors already have a wealth of expertise in teaching in helping bring materials to life, and in creating a stimulating learning environment. This guide is intended to help you do what you already do well and to help make the adjustment to teaching new content a bit easier for you.

Using all these resources, as outlined in this instructor's guide, will help you prepare students to provide hospice and palliative care for individuals experiencing life threatening illness and their families and significant others, through death and bereavement.

How to Use the Instructor's Guide

What topics are covered in the text?

Essentials in Hospice and Palliative Care: A Resource for Nursing Assistants, the text to which this instructor's guide relates, is divided into seven chapters. The first and last chapters focus on the NA – the first on preparing to care, and the last on caring for oneself and continuing to care. The other chapters focus on the dying process, hospice and palliative care, and the dual importance of integrating a palliative approach, and providing physical comfort, psychosocial care, and caregiving in the last days and hours.

Unless otherwise noted, page numbers referenced in this guide relate to the text.

What are the companion resources?

Workbook

The workbook is a competency-based resource designed to help students develop the attitudes, knowledge, and skills for working in hospice and palliative care. It closely follows the text, addressing core concepts and skill development to help students become confident and competent in providing compassionate care for the dying person and family.

Questions in the workbook are referenced in both the instructor's guide and the PowerPoint™ presentations, and are identified by the chapter number and question number (e.g., Ch. 1 Qs 1–3 = Chapter 1 Questions 1 through 3).

Teaching Presentations (PPTs)

Teaching presentations were prepared using Microsoft PowerPoint™ software and throughout this guide are referred to as "PPTs." The PPTs follow the teaching outline, and provide a lecture line for instructors to follow and lecture notes containing suggestions for teaching, activities, and key points to address. I highly recommend that you print the PPTs in what PPT (Microsoft) identifies as the NOTES PAGE format. Using the PPTs and the instructor's guide together will facilitate both your preparation and teaching.

Activities

Activities in the PPTs are also referenced in the instructor's guide. The notes section of the PPTs contain instructions for activities.

Videos

Videos were developed to help you teach about two difficult and very common symptoms: pain and difficult breathing. Another video is titled *Self-Care and Boundaries*. A number of other videos are currently being planned.

Podcasts

The podcasts allow students to hear lecture content outside of classroom time and can deepen discussion, as well as facilitate integration activities during classroom time. Some of you may know this as the "flipped classroom." Podcasts are available on the Life and Death Matters website at http://lifeanddeathmatters.ca.

Podcasts referenced in the instructor's guide are identified by the podcast name and the length of the podcast in minutes and seconds, for example, Hooks – Moving onto Someone Else's Dance Floor . . . 5'54".

How is the Instructor's Guide organized?

Each chapter of the instructor's guide corresponds to the chapter of the same title in the text and contains the components described below.

Learning Outcomes

Learning Outcomes addressed in each chapter are identified in a table at the beginning of each chapter. You may want to summarize or simplify these in order to keep the "end in view."

Teaching Resources

A chapter in the workbook and a PPT presentation correspond to each chapter of the text. The guide also identifies podcasts and videos that relate to the topic. You may want to add other resources, such as local resources, to this list.

Preparation – Instructors

These sections in the instructor's guide identify what you might want to read, review, watch, and listen to as you prepare to teach.

Preparation – Students

Readings, podcasts and questions that you may want to assign to students to help prepare them for class are provided in these sections of the instructor's guide.

Lesson Plan

The lesson plan provides a suggested order for presenting the content to students. Generally, the lesson plan follows the flow of the text and the PPTs. Instructions for the activities mentioned in the lesson plan are located in the NOTES PAGE of the PPT.

Again, I encourage you to print the PPT presentation, in PPT NOTES PAGE format, and assemble the printed pages in a three-ring binder. This will make it easier to use the resources together.

Options for Teaching Hospice and Palliative Care Content in Core Curriculum

There are many ways to teach hospice and palliative care content using these resources. Three options are: 1) teach as a separate module; 2) integrate throughout core curriculum; or 3) a combination, with specific components integrated into core curriculum and a separate module.

Feedback from Instructors suggest that 1) providing resources to students early in the program, and 2) integrating some content into other areas of curriculum, enriches the learning experience. In particular, it is helpful to teach self-reflection early in the program and encourage students to reflect when they come face to face with life-threatening illness, death, loss, and grief in their personal life, classroom discussions, or practicums. Teaching about the dying process early in the program helps students understand that a palliative approach can be integrated early in disease process. Integrating some of the common symptoms into related areas of core curriculum can help people understand disease progression and help decrease the amount of teaching time required for a separate module.

When the content is taught as a separate module, it is helpful to have between 25–30 hours for teaching.

Teaching this content to NAs in continuing education settings

When teaching experienced NAs in a continuing education setting, all of the nine common symptoms should be highlighted. With these students, I tend to start with the introductory content on tools, communication, and palliation, and then address pain, difficult breathing, and decreased appetite and weight loss. I then determine, on the basis of the needs of the group, which symptoms I will address individually and which ones I will link to or dovetail with teaching about the last days and hours of a dying person's life.

Preparing to Care

Learning Outcomes

At the end of this chapter, students will be able to:

1. Reflect on one's personal experiences, beliefs and values regarding death, dying, loss and grief.

2. Explain how personal beliefs and attitudes can impact caregiving.

3. Define therapeutic boundaries and how they affect care of the dying person.

4. Respect spiritual and cultural practices relating to death, dying and after life.

5. Provide emotional support for the dying person and his/her family.

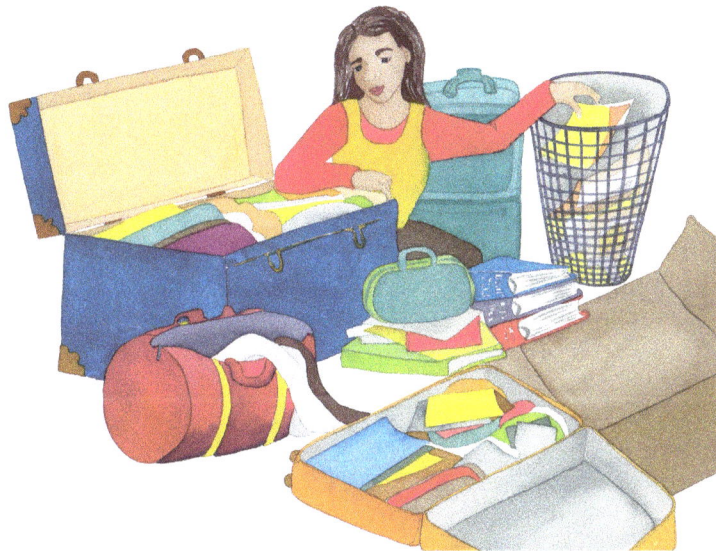

Teaching Resources

Text, workbook, and PPT Ch. 1 Preparing to Care

Podcasts
   a. Self-Awareness . . . . 6'32"
   b. Value of Maintaining a Therapeutic Distance . . . . 6'19"
   c. Phrases to Use . . . . 5'55"
   d. Knowing When You Have Crossed a Boundary onto Someone Else's Dance Floor . . . . 5'54"
   e. Hooks – Moving onto Someone Else's Dance Floor . . . . 5'54"
   f. Our Role in Maintaining Therapeutic Boundaries . . . . 15'35"
   g. Signs That You Are on Someone Else's Dance Floor . . . . 15'13"

Video/DVD: *Self-Care and Boundaries*

Flip chart

Preparation – Instructors

Review the Learning Outcomes to help you focus discussion and learning activities.

1. In the text, read Ch. 1 "Preparing to Care" and the "Loss and Grief" section on p. 134 of Ch. 5 "Providing Psychosocial Care."

2. Review Qs 1–5 in the workbook (consider engaging in the reflective activities yourself).

3. Familiarize yourself with PPT Ch. 1.

4. Listen to the podcast "Self-Awareness."

Preparation – Students

1. In the text, read Ch. 1 "Preparing to Care" and the "Loss and Grief" section on p. 134 of Ch. 5 "Providing Psychosocial Care."

2. Listen to one or more of the following podcasts:
   a. Self-Awareness . . . . 6'32"
   b. Value of Maintaining a Therapeutic Distance . . . . 6'19"
   c. Phrases to Use. . . . . 5'55"

3. Complete Ch. 1 Qs 1–3 in the workbook.

4. Begin the "Preparing to Care" activity (instructions in NOTE PAGE of PPT) by asking students to write reflectively on these two questions:

"What do I know and/or feel about caring for the dying?"

"What do I want to learn, feel and experience about caring for the dying?"

They will be asked to post some or all of their responses to these questions on a flip chart page at the beginning of next class.

Lesson Plan

1. Introducing the Resources

    a. Introduce the text *Essentials in Hospice and Palliative Care: A Resource for Nursing Assistants.*

    b. Introduce the workbook. Explain that attitudes, knowledge, and skills are "competencies" and that each chapter of the workbook has a section that focuses on these competences: the "Understanding Your Beliefs and Baggage" reflective activities are designed to help students clarify or develop awareness and attitudes necessary to work with the dying persons and families; the "Solidifying Concepts" activities are designed to help students develop knowledge; and the "Integrating into Practice" activities help students develop skills.

    c. Consider inviting students to respond to reflective questions by writing in English or their first language, or using mind-maps or art.

    d. Mark reflective questions on the basis of students' participation in the reflection, either through writing, creating mind-maps, or drawing. Ensure that students understand that their reflection will not be marked as either right or wrong.

    e. Introduce the podcasts and provide the links for them. Teach students how to access and listen to the podcasts, or have a student teach the class how to do this. The podcasts provide students with lecture material while they are outside of class, thereby freeing up classroom time for discussion and applying the content in practice.

2. Preparing to Care

    a. Prepare a flip chart to collect answers for the "Preparing to Care" activity

    b. Begin with the "Preparing to Care" activity. Provide students with sticky notes as they enter the class. Instruct them to write their reflections (from homework Preparation – Students Q 4), one reflection per sticky note, and post them to the appropriate flip chart page.

    c. Invite students who are currently having any difficult experiences involving loss, grief, death, or dying to meet with you to explore ways to support them while they are studying this content.

3. Life Is a Journey

    a. Discuss and debrief homework Ch. 1 Qs 2 and 3.

    b. Remind students that the reflective questions will be marked on the basis of their participation in the reflection and their writing or drawing reflections. These questions will not be marked right or wrong.

4. Beliefs and Baggage

    a. Use PPT Ch. 1 and the text to guide discussion.

    b. Watch these videos:
- Packing for a Trip
- Applying the Idea of Baggage to Caregiving

    c. Complete Ch. 1 Q 4 about labeling baggage.

5. Using Reflection to Develop Self-Awareness

a. Continue with PPT Ch. 1.

b. Assign the small group activity "Ways to Develop Self-Awareness." Debrief with the groups upon completion.

c. Complete the small-group activity using Ch. 1 Qs 6 and 7 about self-awareness.

6. Maintaining Therapeutic Boundaries

a. Continue with the PPT Ch. 1 and text, to introduce the concept of maintaining therapeutic boundaries. This may be a new skill for some or all students. Some may find that maintaining therapeutic boundaries is not congruent with their cultural values and ways of being in the community. Listening to all the related podcasts may help students develop a greater understanding of why maintaining therapeutic boundaries is important both for the people they care for and themselves.

b. Assign the "Understanding Boundaries" activity included in the PPT.

c. Listen and discuss the podcast "Knowing When You Have Crossed a Boundary onto Someone Else's Dance Floor."

d. Complete Ch. 1 Q 5.

Understanding the Dying Process

Learning Outcomes

At the end of this chapter, students will be able to:

1. Describe the four patterns of decline that illustrate the dying processes.

2. Understand the concept of providing emotional support for the dying person and their family.

3. Discuss the impact of life-threatening illnesses and life transitions on a dying person and the family and on the nursing assistant.

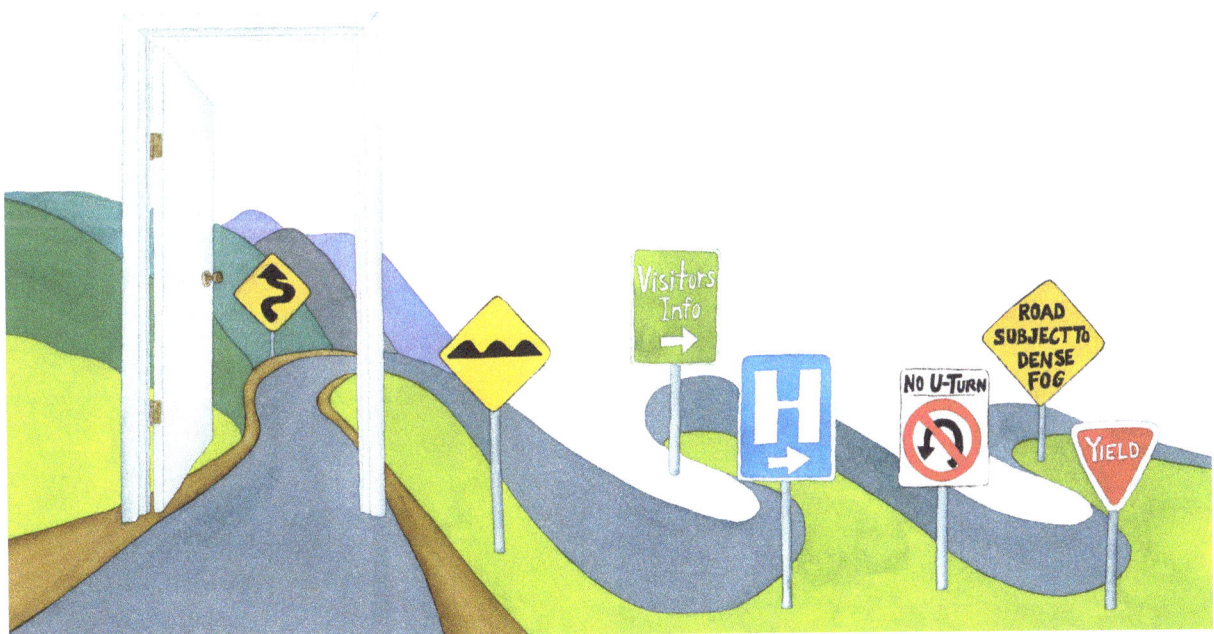

Teaching Resources

Text, workbook, and PPT Ch. 2 Understanding the Dying Process

Podcast

    Scenarios in Hospice Palliative Care with Bob . . . . 16'44"

Preparation – Instructors

Review the Learning Outcomes to help you focus discussion and learning activities.

1. Read Ch. 2 "Understanding the Dying Process" and Ch. 5 page 126 "Supporting Choice, Control, and Independence."

2. Review the questions in Ch. 2 in the workbook, and familiarize yourself with PPT Ch. 2.

Preparation – Students

1. Read Ch. 2, "Understanding the Dying Process" and Ch. 5 page 126 "Supporting Choice, Control, and Independence," then complete Ch. 2 Q 1.

Lesson Plan

1. People Have Never Died Like This

a. Use PPT Ch. 2 and the text to guide discussion.

b. View the *Unprecedented – Common Patterns of Dying* video.

c. Discuss the difference between the process of dying now in comparison to how people died in the past. Unlike in past centuries, nowadays the process of dying occurs over a longer period of time, people require help for a longer period of time, and fewer caregivers are available to provide care. How will the changes in the way people are dying affect caregiving now and in the future? How will this affect students' abilities to find work in this field of caregiving?

d. Students may want to answer Ch. 2 Q 3 at this time.

2. Patterns of Dying

a. Continue with PPT Ch. 2 and the text to guide discussion.

b. Consider the stories in the text, as well as your personal and professional experiences and the personal experiences of students.

c. Complete the "Patterns of Dying" (Ch. 2 Q 4) exercise as an individual or group activity.

d. Review and discuss the answers to Ch. 2. Q 1 (My preferences about dying).

e. Review and discuss the answers to Ch. 2 Q 2 (Preferences for a loved one's dying). Discuss why it is important for the dying person and family to have this information in order to make decisions. This is a recurring theme throughout the text.

f. Discuss why it is important for people to talk about issues related to death, dying, medical decisions, and so on. Encourage students to start discussions with their families about end of life. If a holiday is approaching, and students are gathering with family over the holidays, you may want students to read the "Advance Care Planning" section in Ch. 5 "Providing Psychosocial Care" and encourage them to address these topics with their loved ones.

3. The Dying Process

a. Emphasize the importance of supporting the dying person to help maintain their ability to make choices. This also is a recurring theme throughout the resources.

b. As a group, address Ch. 2 Qs 5 and 6, and have students complete remaining questions in the workbook.

c. Discuss the metaphor that compares caregiving with running a race (see p. 23 in the text).

Integrating a Palliative Approach into Caregiving 3

Learning Outcomes

At the end of this chapter students will be able to:

1. Understand and describe the concepts of palliative, hospice and end-of-life care.

2. Discuss the philosophy, principles and practices associated with providing palliative care.

3. Differentiate between sympathy and empathy.

4. Identify ways to create a safe, nurturing place, by understanding how verbal and non-verbal communication may be shaped by cultural practices, identifying common barriers to communication and using techniques to minimize their impact in patient-nursing assistant relationships.

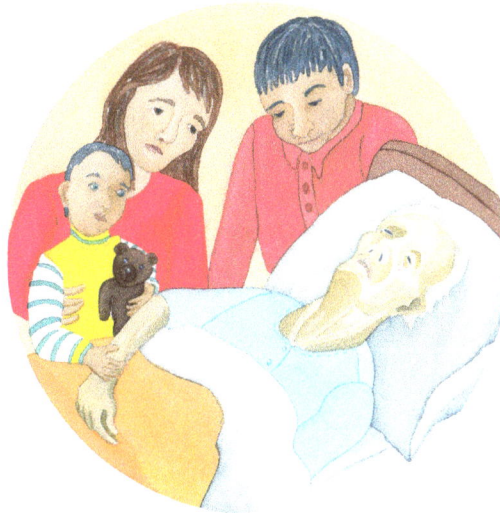

Teaching Resources

Text, workbook, and PPT Ch. 3 Integrating a Palliative Approach into Caregiving

Podcasts

    a. Roadblocks to Communication – Giving Praise . . . . 10'28"

    b. Roadblocks to Communication – Giving Advice . . . . 15'52"

    c. Roadblocks to Communication – Giving Reassurance . . . . 10'58"

    d. Roadblocks to Communication – Using Empathic Listening Lead-ins in Hospice and Palliative Care . . 5'24"

Preparation – Instructors

Review the Learning Outcomes to help you focus discussion and learning activities.

1. Read Ch. 3 "Integrating a Palliative Approach into Caregiving" in the text and review the questions in the workbook.

2. Familiarize yourself with PPT Ch. 3.

3. Consider the common roadblocks to communication. Prepare examples to illustrate each roadblock, or prepare to demonstrate each roadblock.

Preparation – Students

1. Read Ch. 3 "Integrating a Palliative Approach into Caregiving" in the text.

2. Complete Ch. 3 Qs 1–3 in the workbook.

Lesson Plan

1. The Beginning of Better Care for the Dying

Use PPT Ch. 3 and text to guide discussion on the principles of hospice and palliative care and applying them when caregiving early in the disease process.

2. A Palliative Approach

    a. Define the key concept of a palliative approach, and discuss the rationale for integrating a palliative approach into caregiving.

        i. Explain the importance of integrating a palliative approach early in the disease process, for people with any life-threatening illness, across all care settings.

        ii. Debrief and discuss students' answers to Ch. 3 Q 1 (principles of hospice and palliative care and integrating it early in the dying process).

        iii. Emphasize the points made in the text box " 'Palliative' Describes a Type of Care" on p. 31 in the text.

    b. Assign Ch. 3. Q 4 (crossword puzzle).

    c. Invite students to complete workbook Ch. 3 Qs 5–8 during class discussion (or assign as homework).

3. Terms Used in Hospice and Palliative Care

    a. Identify which terms students will need to know in your area.

    b. Emphasize how to use the term "palliative" correctly.

4. Health Care Team

a. Continue with PPT Ch. 3, using the text as a reference.

b. Discuss the value of all team members, including and especially NAs.

c. Discuss how the text attempts to honor the role of the NA and the incredible contributions made by NAs.

d. Emphasize the need for the NA to participate on the team, to share observations, and to advocate as needed for the dying person and family.

e. Identify the ways that NAs support and integrate a palliative approach.

5. "Good Death, Bad Death"

a. As a group, discuss Ch. 3 Q 13. You may want to use a flip chart to discuss and record students' responses about what is a good or a bad death for them.

Emphasize the variety of answers and how it helps reveal that a good death is unique for each person. Encourage input from students on how to adapt care to help take into account the individual preferences written on the flip chart.

b. Discuss ways to support dignity, and as a group discuss the "dignity question" on p. 42 of the text.

c. Assign Ch. 3 Q 14 on the "Dignity Question" for students to complete in class.

6. How NAs Provide Support: Creating a Nurturing Place

a. Continue with PPT Ch. 3, using the text as a reference.

b. Listen to podcasts "Roadblocks to Communication" in class or assign as out-of-class work.

c. Discuss the ways that NAs provide support by avoiding roadblocks to communication, offering a compassionate presence, and supporting dignity.

d. Discuss behaviors that help to create a safe and nurturing place.

e. Identify common roadblocks:

   i. Discuss answers to workbook Ch. 3 Qs 2 and 3.

   ii. Share examples or demonstrate how well-intentioned people can actually block communication when they minimize the problem; offer false reassurance, praise, platitudes, or sympathy; attempt to fix problems; and judge or label people.

f. Ask students to complete workbook Ch. 3 Qs 9, 10, 15, and 16.

g. Ask students to work in pairs to role-play the scenario in Ch. 3 Q 12.

h. Discuss ways to provide a compassionate presence.

4 Increasing Physical Comfort

Learning Outcomes

At the end of this chapter students will be able to:

1. Observe and record the dying person's vital signs according to the direction of the plan of care* and using identified communication tools e.g., flow sheets, graphs, etc.

2. Use pain scales to record the dying person's pain responses.

3. Seek feedback from the dying person as to what their comfort needs are and their responses to comfort management techniques.

4. Observe and report relevant dying person's information, e.g., changes in person's status and/or service to appropriate members of the inter-professional team.

5. Identify and use appropriate medical terminology.

6. Identify and discuss methods of recording and reporting client care information.

7. Discuss the person's plan of care/service plan* as a communication tool.

8. Discuss the role of advocacy for the dying person, their families and significant others.

PowerPoint™ presentations (PPTs) for Chapter 4

Ch. 4 "Increasing Physical Comfort" identifies tools and strategies to help increase physical comfort for the dying person. It also discusses comfort measures for NAs to use to support the family. Because there is a wealth of information to teach in this section, the PPTs are divided into these 10 separate presentations.

Ch. 4A: Tools and Communication for Physical Comfort
Ch. 4B: Principles of Palliation
Ch. 4C: Pain
Ch. 4D: Difficult Breathing
Ch. 4E: Decreased Appetite and Weight Loss
Ch. 4F: Changes in Bowel and Bladder Function
Ch. 4G: Dehydration
Ch. 4H: Delirium
Ch. 4I: Fatigue
Ch. 4J: Mouth Discomfort
Ch. 4K: Nausea and Vomiting

I recommend that you start by teaching Ch. 4A Tools and Communication for Physical Comfort and Ch. 4B Principles of Palliation, followed by the high priority topics Ch. 4B: Pain, Ch. 4C: Difficult Breathing and Ch. 4D: Decreased Appetite and Weight Loss. If you have limited time to teach this content, and are not able to discuss ALL the common symptoms, I suggest teaching at least these three symptoms in detail.

The remaining symptoms can be taught within related areas of core curriculum and then recapped during a separate module. Consider these teaching options.

Changes in Bowel and Bladder function could be introduced by saying, "We have talked about bowel and bladder issues as a person is aging. Let's look at the specific challenges that people experience when they have a life-threatening illness and when they are actively dying."

Decreased Appetite and Weight Loss and Dehydration can be introduced when discussing nutrition, and then discussed again during a separate module.

Delirium can be introduced when discussing dementia, delirium and depression, and then reintroduced again when teaching about last days and hours.

Fatigue may be addressed when discussing the individual's need for control, emphasizing how important it is to have choices and to prioritize activities when people experience profound fatigue. Fatigue can also be addressed when discussing decreased mobility, and when identifying strategies to support people whose fatigue means they need to choose between having the energy to walk to the dining room, or having the energy to eat their food. A comfort strategy might be to use the wheel chair to get to the dining room to eat.

Mouth Discomfort can be taught with mouth care, and then again when discussing last days and hours.

And finally, Nausea and Vomiting may be taught when discussing gastrointestinal issues, and then revisited during this module.

When revisiting these symptoms during the module, use the information in the text and questions in the workbook to help students integrate the content.

Chapter 4A: Tools and Communication for Physical Comfort

Teaching Resources

Text, workbook, and PPT Ch. 4A: Tools and Communication for Physical Comfort

Flip chart and paper

Preparation – Instructors

Review the Learning Outcomes to help you focus discussion and learning activities.

1. Read pp. 49–57, 103 (PAINAD) and 105 (Body Map) in Ch. 4 "Increasing Physical Comfort" in the text.

2. Review the related workbook questions, and familiarize yourself with PPT Ch. 4A.

Preparation – Students

1. Read pp. 49–57 in Ch. 4 "Increasing Physical Comfort" in the text.

2. Complete Ch. 4 Q 1 and Q 2 (crossword puzzle) in the workbook.

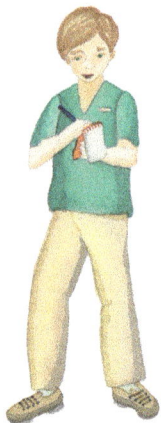

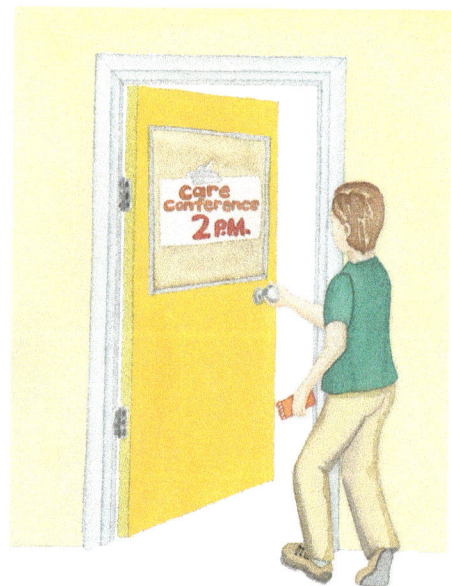

Lesson Plan

1. Tools for Gathering Information

    a. Debrief students on Ch. 4 Q 1.

    b. Discuss why NAs are ideally positioned to gather information about the dying person.

2. Palliative Performance Scale (PPS)

    a. Use PPT Ch. 4A and the text to guide discussion.

    b. Complete the activity "Using the PPS".

    c. Discuss how the PPS can be used as a tool for communicating with the care team, and how using the PPS can help the team understand what type of care the dying person and their family may require.

    d. Complete Ch. 4. Qs 3–5.

3. List of Sample Questions

    a. Discuss the List of Sample Questions, which are adapted from the "Symptom Assessment Acronym – OPQRSTUV," a tool that health care teams use for symptom assessment. While assessing a person may not be part of the role of NAs, they can gather information to provide to the health care team.

    b. When possible, NAs might explore all the sample questions with the person. Students may want to highlight the following four questions, as they identify what, when, how severe it is and how to help.
        a. What is happening? What is wrong?
        b. When did it start?
        c. Can you rate is on a scale?
        d. What makes it better or worse?

    Emphasize that the NA might want to consider how many questions they should ask before they begin.

4. Other Tools – Pain Assessment in Advanced Dementia (PAINAD) and Body Map

    a. Identify the role of the PAINAD and Body Map tools in gathering information. Details of these tools are in the text on pp. 103 and 105 respectively.

5. Communicating with the Team

    a. Continue with PPS Ch. 4A and focus discussion on the characteristics of good recording and reporting.

    b. Discuss the importance of establishing relationships within the care team, and the need to communicate information clearly and concisely in order to be heard.

    c. Complete the "Reporting Appropriate Information" activity.

6. Advocating

    a. Use the PPT Ch. 4A and text to discuss ways that an NA can advocate for the dying person and their family.

    b. Identify tips for advocating.

    c. Complete Ch. 4 Q 6 in the workbook.

Chapter 4B: Principles of Palliation

Teaching Resources

Text, workbook, and PPT Ch. 4B: Principles of Palliation

Podcasts

    a. Principles for Managing Symptoms in Hospice and Palliative Care . . . . 9'55'
    b. Hospice and Palliative Care Principles for Using Medications to Manage Symptoms. . . . . 9'14"
    c. Basket of Comfort Measures . . . . 19'25"

Flip chart and paper

Preparation – Instructors

Review the Learning Outcomes to help you focus discussion and learning activities.

1. In the text, read pp. 58–64 and 108–116 in Ch. 4 "Increasing Physical Comfort."

2. Familiarize yourself with PPT Ch. 4B.

3. Listen to these podcasts:
    a. Principles for Managing Symptoms in Hospice and Palliative Care . . . . 9'55"
    b. Hospice and Palliative Care Principles for Using Medications to Manage Symptoms . . . . 9'14"
    c. Basket of Comfort Measures . . . . 19'25"

Preparation – Students

1. In the text, read pp. 58–64 and 113–116 in Ch. 4 "Increasing Physical Comfort."

2. Listen to these podcasts:
    a. Principles for Managing Symptoms in Hospice and Palliative Care . . . . 9'55"
    b. Hospice and Palliative Care Principles for Using Medications to Manage Symptoms . . . . 9'14"
    c. Basket of Comfort Measures . . . . 19'25"

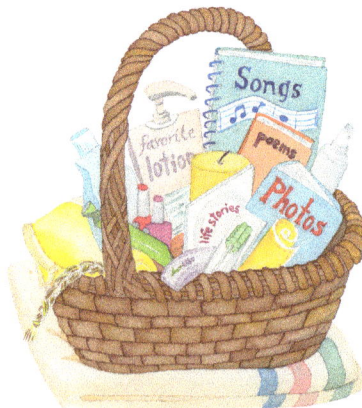

Lesson Plan

1. Principles of Palliation

a. Follow PPT Ch. 4A and the text as a guide.

b. Complete the Principles of Palliation activity.

The goal of this activity is to help students understand why, in hospice and palliative care, medications are given regularly, around the clock, and doses are increased or decreased according to the person's needs and goals of care. This is their opportunity to ask questions and express concerns about how medications are used in palliative care. When students are in the clinical setting it is not appropriate to discuss their concerns about medications with the dying person and family present. It is also inappropriate for students to give advice about medications to the dying person and family.

c. Remind students that they are not responsible for ordering or dispensing medications to manage symptoms, but they are going to hear dying people and family members express concerns and ask questions about medications. It is appropriate for the NA to respond to such questions with "that is a good question" and communicate concerns to the nurse or health care team. Remind students that it is inappropriate for them to give advice about medications.

d. Complete Ch. 4 Qs 7 and 8 in the workbook.

2. Using Opioids to Manage Symptoms

a. Continue with PPT Ch. 4B and discuss using opioids to manage symptoms.

b. Identify the common fears people have about using opioids, and discuss ways to help when the family expresses fears or asks questions about their use.

3. Basket of Comfort Measures

a. Using PPT Ch. 4B and the text, identify ways that non-pharmacological comfort measures can support the dying person.

b. Discuss the guidelines for using comfort measures.

c. Post a flip chart page and have students add their ideas for comfort measures from their own lives.

Pain

Teaching Resources

Pages 101–114 and Appendix A (pp. 205–210) in the text, Ch. 4 Qs 22–25 (marking sheet for Q 23 role-plays is on pp. 60–61 in the workbook), and PPT Ch. 4C: Pain

Flip chart page and sticky notes or marker pens

Materials/Equipment:

    a. Pillows for positioning activity
    b. Props for role play

1. Podcasts
    a. Using Medications to Manage Symptoms . . . . 8'15"
    b. Managing Pain in Hospice and Palliative Care . . . . 15'15"
    c. Introduction to Understanding Pain . . . . 15'20"
    d. Assessing Pain in Hospice and Palliative Care . . . . 23'00"

Preparation – Instructors

1. Read pp. 101–114 in the text and familiarize yourself with PPT Ch. 4C and Ch. 4 Qs 22–25 in the workbook.

2. Materials and Equipment
Pillows and beds/flat surfaces to demonstrate and practice positioning for comfort.
Props for role play

Preparation – Students

1. Read pp. 101–114 in the text and complete the "Reflection Activity on Different Types of Pain" on p. 107. For each different type of pain, write words to describe how the pain feels. If you haven't experienced one or more of the three types of pain, ask your family, friends, or colleagues about their experiences of pain and how they would describe it.

2. Depending on the time available, consider having students listen to the podcasts either in the class or as homework.

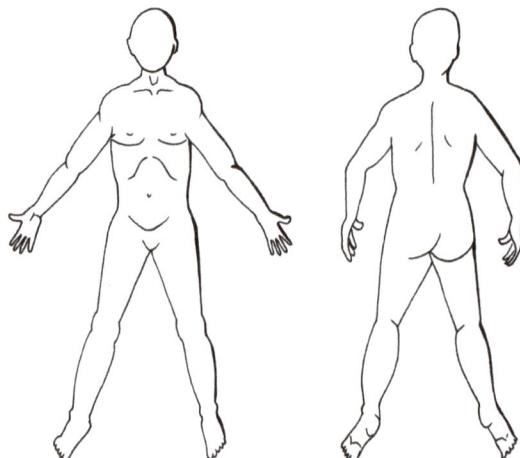

Lesson Plan

1. Pain

    a. Use PPT Ch. 4C.

    b. Review the tools for gathering information.

    c. Complete the classroom portion of the "Reflection Activity on Different Types of Pain" p. 107 by collecting student's descriptions of pain on the flip chart page.

    d. Discuss: How is pain a whole person experience?

        i. Watch the video *Introduction to Managing Pain*.

        ii. Debrief the video and any questions or concerns that NA students might have about pain, pain management, and the use of medication.

2. Comfort Measures

    a. Engage in the "Positioning for Comfort" activity.

    b. Discuss ways to support a person in pain.

    c. Identify ways to engage the family in providing comfort.

    d. Discuss the comfort basket and ways to enhance comfort.

3. Role Plays

    a. Have students work through some or all of the role-plays, Ch. 4 Qs 22 and 23 in the workbook. Use props if available to enhance the learning experience.

    b. Complete Ch. 4 Qs 24 and 25.

4. Assign podcasts for students to listen to either in the class or as homework, as time permits.

Difficult Breathing

Teaching Resources

Text, workbook, and PPT Ch. 4D: Difficult Breathing

Materials/equipment:

a. Three disposable straws per student for the dyspnea exercise (Ch. 4 Q 17 in the workbook)

b. Bed(s) and pillows for demonstrating and practicing positioning to improve breathing

Video/DVD: *Dyspnea – the Feeling of Breathlessness*

Preparation – Instructors

1. Read pp. 85–89 in the text, and familiarize yourself with the dyspnea exercise (Ch. 4 Q 17 in the workbook) and PPT Ch. 4D.

Preparation – Students

1. Read pp. 85–89 in the text.

Lesson Plan

1. Difficult Breathing

a. Use PPT Ch. 4D and text to focus a discussion about difficult breathing.

b. Discuss why it is important to know that difficult breathing is what a person says it is—it is subjective and cannot be measured.

c. Complete the Dyspnea Exercise in Workbook Ch. 4 Q 17 or in the video *Dyspnea – The Feeling of Breathlessness*.

d. Have students complete Ch. 4 Qs 17a–c. You may want to post a flip chart page on the wall on which students can write their reflections. The hope is that the dyspnea exercise will increase students' understanding of how difficult this symptom can be.

e. Watch the video *Dyspnea – the Feeling of Breathlessness*.

2. Comfort Measures

a. Invite students to participate in the activity "Coaching Breathing." Follow the instructions in the Text pp. 87, 88.

b. Have students complete Ch. 4. Q 18.

c. Demonstrate ways to position a person who is experiencing difficult breathing. After the demonstration, have students work in pairs or small groups to practice positioning one another. If this is not possible in the classroom, invite the instructors in the lab or the practicum to assist with this demonstration.

d. Identify three comfort measures to help a person with difficult breathing – as prevention, in the moment, and as disease progresses. Discuss how NAs might support the family.

3. Palliation

a. Discuss the use of opioids for people with difficult breathing.

Decreased Appetite and Weight Loss

Teaching Resources

Text, workbook, and PPT Ch. 4E: Decreased Appetite and Weight Loss

Podcast

Anorexia and Cachexia in Hospice and Palliative Care . . . . 23'04"

Preparation – Instructors

1. Read pp. 68–73 in Ch. 4 "Increasing Physical Comfort" in the text and review Qs 13 and 14 in the workbook.

2. Familiarize yourself with PPT Ch. 4E.

3. Listen to the podcast "Anorexia and Cachexia in Hospice and Palliative Care."

Preparation – Students

1. Read pp. 68–73 in Ch. 4 "Increasing Physical Comfort" in the text.

2. Write reflectively on the statement "Food is more than just fuel for the body." What does food mean to you, your culture, and your family? What role has food played in your life?

Lesson Plan

1. Decreased Appetite and Weight Loss

a. Use PPT Ch. 4E and the text.

b. Debrief students on their reflections about "Food is more than just fuel for the body" to develop their understanding of the different roles that food plays in people's lives.

c. Discuss possible causes of decreased appetite and weight loss in dying people and these symptoms are common.

d. Explain to students that decreased appetite and involuntary weight loss can be very stressful for the dying person's family and can cause great conflict between the family and front line caregivers.

e. Define anorexia and cachexia.

f. Discuss ways to approach conversations about decreased appetite and weight loss with the person.

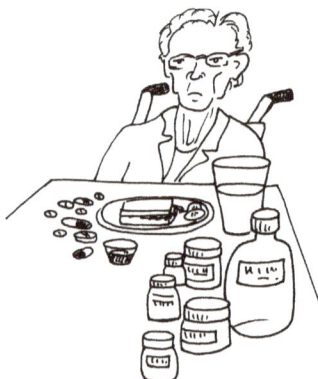

2. **Profound Truths of Nutrition**

   a. Complete the "What Do We Eat?" activity in the PPTs.

   b. Discuss the "Profound Truths of Nutrition" on p. 72 in the text.

   c. Complete Ch. 4 Q 13 in the workbook.

3. **Anorexia and Cachexia**

   a. Discuss characteristics of anorexia and cachexia (Text pg. 72, 73). Have students define anorexia and cachexia. It is important that they understand that this is the specific type of anorexia dying people experience.

   b. Assign the podcast "Anorexia and Cachexia in Hospice and Palliative Care" for class time or homework.

4. **Comfort Measures**

   a. Identify comfort measures to use for the dying person in the moment, later in their disease process, and for the family.

Optional Activities

1. **What Food Means to My Family**

   As an alternative activity, students could create poster presentations on "What Food Means to My Family" or "How Food Intake Changes across the Lifespan," using magazines and other image sources and poster boards. This activity might help students understand the normal changes associated with aging, the increasing struggle to eat that people have when they are sick, and the stress the family experiences when they witness their loved one eating less.

2. **Discussing Truths about Nutrition**

   Depending on the time available, you may want to divide students into small groups to discuss each of the points in the "Profound Truths of Nutrition" text box on p. 72 in the text. Have students brainstorm about the following:

   a. Ways to discuss the truths of nutrition during daily conversations, as a fact of life.

   b. Ways to support the family and help family members nurture the dying person when their food intake declines.

3. **Anorexia and Cachexia in Hospice and Palliative Care**

   It may be helpful to listen to the podcast "Anorexia and Cachexia in Hospice and Palliative Care" to understand these two symptoms and develop new ways of explaining them to the family. This podcast which is based on current research helps people to understand the normal changes in the dying process.

The Other Common Symptoms (in addition to pain, decreasing appetite and weight loss, and dyspnea)

1. Invite students to work together to complete the Ch. 4 workbook questions related to these common symptoms:

   Ch. 4F: Bowel and bladder . . . . Q 12

   Ch. 4G: Dehydration . . . . Q 15

   Ch. 4H: Delirium. . . . . Q 16

   Ch. 4I: Fatigue . . . . Q 19

   Ch. 4J: Mouth discomfort . . . . Q 20

   Ch. 4K: Nausea and vomiting . . . . Q 21

2. Have students listen to these excellent podcasts about dehydration:

   a. The Challenges of Dehydration in Hospice and Palliative Care. . . . . 12'17"

   b. Dehydration and Decreased Fluid Intake in Hospice and Palliative Care (role-play). . . . . .19'54"

3. For each of the common symptoms, have students identify three comfort measures to support the dying person and family.

4. Discuss the role of the NA in helping the person manage common symptoms.

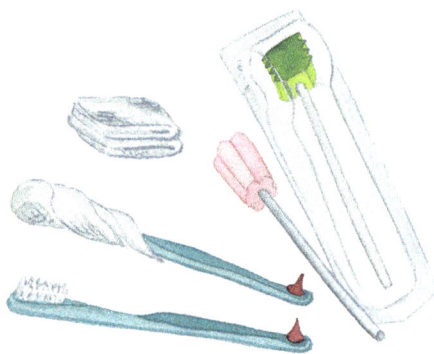

Providing Psychosocial Care

5

Learning Outcomes

At the end of this chapter students will be able to:

1. Provide emotional support for the dying person and their family.

2. Understand and explain the importance of maintaining choice, control and independence for the dying person and ways for PSWs to support these options.

3. Identify ways to communicate the dying person's choices to the team.

4. Explain the importance and ways of respecting the person's rights with respect to end-of-life care.

5. Understand the differences and complexities when dying with dementia.

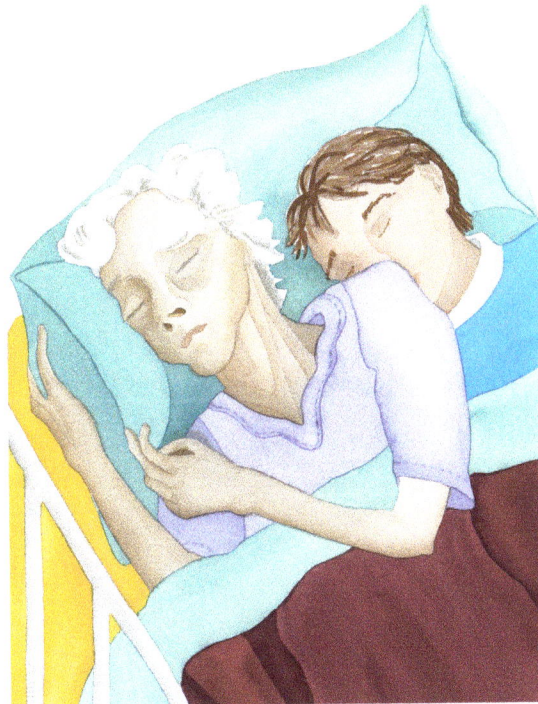

Teaching Resources

Text, workbook, and PPT Ch. 5 Providing Psychosocial Care

Podcasts (choose those that are appropriate for your students):
    a. Death Is a Series of Losses . . . . 11'34"
    b. Common Emotions Associated with Losses in Hospice and Palliative Care . . . . 12'35"
    c. How Are Loss and Grief with Dementia Different? . . . . 11'39"
    d. Psychosocial Perspective – the Holistic Approach, Part 1 . . . . 20'30"
    e. What Defines an Appropriate Death in Hospice and Palliative Care? . . . . 13'20"
    f. Pre-Death 101 – How we can Prepare for Dying with Hospice Palliative Care . . . . 6'46"

Preparation – Instructors

1. Read Ch. 5 "Providing Psychosocial Care" and familiarize yourself with workbook activities and the PPT Ch. 5.

2. Listen to these podcasts:
    a. Psychosocial Perspective – the Holistic Approach, Part 1 . . . . 20'30"
    b. What Defines an Appropriate Death in Hospice and Palliative Care? . . . . 13'20"
    c. Pre-Death 101 – How we can Prepare for Dying with Hospice and Palliative Care . . . . 6'46"

Preparation – Students

1. Read Ch. 5 "Providing Psychosocial Care" in the text before class, answer Ch. 5 Qs 1 and 2 in the workbook, and consider the questions related to advance care planning on p. 130 in the text.

Lesson Plan

Debrief on the homework assignment regarding their readings and responses to the questions about advance care planning.

1. Transitions

    a. Use PPT Ch. 5 and the text.

    b. Discuss the ways the NA's role changes as the dying person's status changes.

2. Sharing Information

    a. During class, play the podcast "Pre-death 101 – How we can Prepare for Dying with Hospice Palliative Care."

    b. Discuss why preparing for death is helpful.

    c. Identify ways for NAs to be supportive during transitions.

3. Dying with Dementia

Most NAs will at some point care for people who are dying with or from dementia. The short summary on pp. 124–125 highlights some of what we don't know and some of what we do know about dying with dementia. This content is important so please take time to cover it. You may want to include dovetail some of this information into the section on the program when you discuss dementias in more depth.

a. Continue with PPT Ch. 5 and the text as guides.

b. Identify differences in dying with dementia. Have students follow the discussion while referring to the text pp. 124–125, to learn about the specific challenges experienced by the dying person and the family when the person is dying with dementia.

4. Supporting Control, Choice and Independence

a. Continue with the PPT.

b. Complete Ch. 5 Q 3 with the students, which will help them examine their own responses to loss as well as their desire for control, choice and independence.

c. Discuss the issues in Ch. 5 Q 4 in the workbook and complete this together. This might raise discussions of ethics as well as the topic of control, choice and desire for independence.

5. Advance Care Planning

a. Debrief answers to the homework assignment about advance care planning on p. 130 in the text.

b. Continue with PPT Ch. 5.

c. Assign students Ch. 5 Qs 6–8.

6. Loss and Grief

a. Continue with PPT Ch. 5.

b. Refer to the "Basic Truths about Loss and Grief" section on p. 134 in the text.

c. Discuss why denial may be a coping strategy for some people (or perhaps for all people some of the time).

d. Identify ways the NA can support people experiencing loss and grief.

e. Have students complete Q 5 and Qs 10–12 in the workbook. Debrief the answers in class.

f. Have students complete Ch. 5 Q 9 (crossword puzzle) in class or assign it as homework.

Optional Activity

Transitions in Dying

Ask students to work alone or in groups to create a visual project that presents the transitions in dying, the PPS levels, the changes in the roles of the dying person and the family, and the different roles the NA plays in each transition. The goal of this project is to help students identify and remember their different roles in these times of transition.

Caring in the Last Days and Hours

6

Learning Outcomes

At the end of this chapter students will be able to:

1. Understand the importance of developing a plan for time of death.

2. Know the importance of rituals and traditions in death.

3. Recognize physical changes and ways to support the dying person and the family in the last days and hours.

4. Identify ways to support the family and care for the body following death.

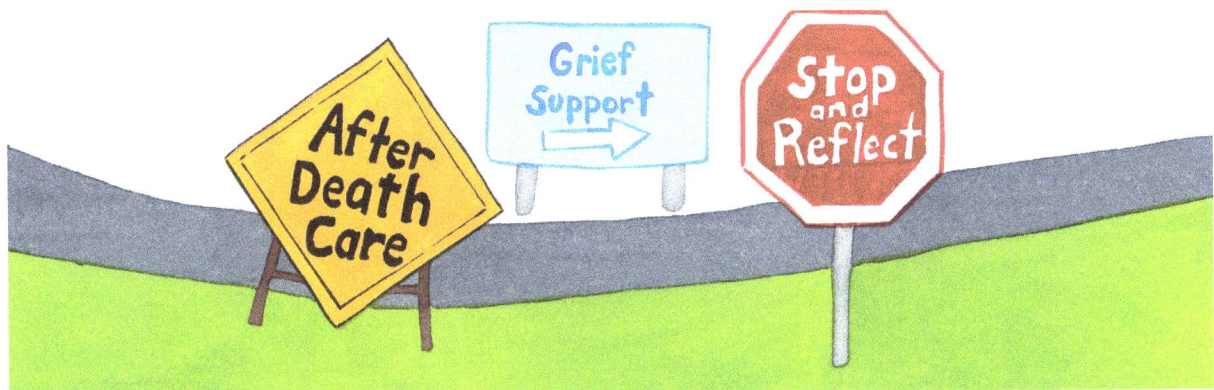

Teaching Resources

Text, workbook, and PPT Ch. 6 Caring in the Last Days and Hours

Flip chart paper and pens or sticky notes

Podcasts:

    a. Changes in Last Days and Hours – Introduction and Drowsiness . . . . 16'19"

    b. Changes in Last Days and Hours – Decreased Intake . . . . 22'48"

    c. Changes in Last Days and Hours – Confusion and Restlessness . . . . 20'07"

    d. Changes in Last Days and Hours – Breathing . . . . 12'03"

    e. Changes in Last Days and Hours – Skin Color . . . . .18'50"

Preparation – Instructors

    a. Read Ch. 6 "Caring in the Last Days and Hours" in the text.

    b. Familiarize yourself with the workbook and PPT Ch. 6.

Preparation – Students

    a. Read Ch. 6 "Caring in the Last Days and Hours" in the text and complete Ch. 6 Qs 1 and 2 in the workbook.

Lesson Plan

1. Preparing to Care

    a. Debrief homework questions.

    b. Use the text and PPT Ch. 6 to guide discussion.

    c. Discuss ways that the health care team can help prepare the family to care for the dying person in the last days and hours. What is the NA's role?

2. Physical Changes and Psychosocial Implications

    a. Emphasize that not every person experiences every change and that the changes do not occur in any particular order.

    b. Discuss why it is important for the family to understand the changes and the potential meaning of the changes.

    c. Use the text and PPT Ch. 6 to identify the changes, and discuss comfort measures for each of them. Students may want to complete Ch. 6 Q 3 in the workbook during discussion of each physical change.

    d. Invite students to listen to the podcasts on Changes in Last Days and Hours, to develop their understanding of the changes and the psychosocial implications of the changes.

3. When Death Occurs

    a. Identify what to expect to see when the person has died.

    b. Invite students to complete Ch. 6 Q 4.

4. When Death Is Expected

a. Identify what the NA can do after a person dies if there is a care plan and a signed DNR.

b. Discuss Ch. 6 Qs 5 and 6, and answer students' questions as necessary, so that students clearly understand this concept.

c. Refer to the text p. 176 and review how to care for the body after death.

d. Emphasize that the NA is to follow the family's lead in terms of rituals. Discuss ways that the NA can invite family to discuss rituals by asking neutral questions. You may want to post a flip chart page to the wall and have students write on it suggestions for ways to invite discussion with families.

e. Answer Ch. 6 Q 8 on supporting rituals and traditions that are different from one's own.

f. Have students work in small groups to complete Ch. 6 Q 10a.

5. Supporting the Family

a. Discuss ways to support the family after the death occurs and how this might change in a variety of care settings.

b. Have students complete Ch. 6 Q 7, 10a about how to support the family after the death of their loved one.

6. Debriefing with Staff

a. Continue with PPT Ch. 6.

b. Identify ways for NAs to debrief after a death.

7. Preparing to Transfer the Body

a. Review care that is commonly provided before transferring a body on p. 185 in the text. Remind students that they must follow agency or facility policies on how to prepare the body for transport.

8. The Home Funeral Movement

a. Briefly discuss how funerals have changed and the emergence of new funeral providers.

Note: Ch. 6 Q 11 is to be completed when students are doing a practicum.

7

Caring for *You!*

Learning Outcomes

At the end of this chapter students will be able to:

1. Define compassion fatigue and know when self-care strategies are necessary.

2. Understand methods of self-care and the importance of using these methods when caring for the dying.

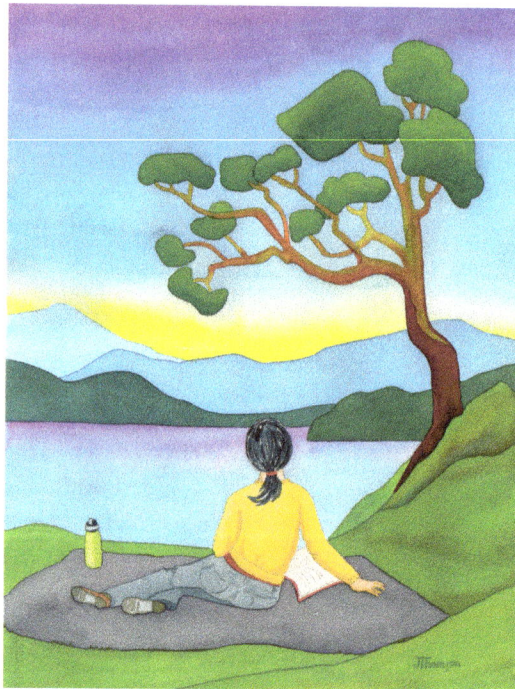

Teaching Resources

Text, workbook, and PPT Ch. 7 Caring for You!

Preparation – Instructors

Read Ch. 7, "Caring for You!" and familiarize yourself with the workbook and PPT Ch. 7.

Preparation – Students

Read Ch. 7, "Caring for You!" in the text and complete Q 1.

Lesson Plan

1. **Providing Care for the Dying will Change You**

    a. Debrief the homework question Ch. 7 Q 1.

    b. Follow the lecture line in PPT Ch. 7 and use the text as a guide.

2. **Self-Care – Buffering the Effects of Caregiving**

    a. Discuss why self-care is important for people who care for the dying.

    b. Identify strategies for self-care.

3. **Checking In: Signs of Compassion Fatigue**

    a. Using Mathieu's chart on pp. 194–195 in the text, discuss the key points for identifying compassion fatigue.

    b. Have students complete Ch. 7 Q 3 about compassion fatigue. You may want to use this as a homework assignment after showing PPT Ch. 7.

4. **Self-Care Strategies for Caregivers**

    a. Assign students Ch. 7 Q 2.

    b. Follow the text and PPT Ch. 7, and discuss the self-care strategies.

    c. Ask students to identify strategies that they might consider trying.

    d. Assign students Ch. 7 Qs 4 and 5.

5. **Reflection**

    a. Complete Ch. 7 Qs 6 and 7.

www.ingramcontent.com/pod-product-compliance
Lightning Source LLC
Chambersburg PA
CBHW050040220326
41599CB00044B/7237